MW00569300

10-MINUTE WORKOUTS

FOR PEOPLE WITH DIABETES

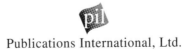

Publications International, Ltd.

Front cover image: Shutterstock.com

Interior photography: Christopher Hiltz

Consultant and fitness model: Katie Morgan

Louis Weber, CEO
Publications International, Ltd.
7373 North Cicero Avenue
Lincolnwood, Illinois 60712

ISBN: 978-1-4508-9632-0

Manufactured in U.S.A.

8 7 6 5 4 3 2 1

TABLE OF CONTENTS

INTRODUCTION

Anyone who's been diagnosed with diabetes or prediabetes by their health care provider has probably gotten the recommendation to make some lifestyle changes. This thought can be daunting. In some ways it's easier to imagine taking medication than it is to imagine blocking out time to exercise each day, or thinking carefully, every meal, about food intake. But committing to making those lifestyle changes can be empowering instead of limiting. You'll have the reward of seeing your blood sugar levels drop and the knowledge that you're playing a part in maintaining your health.

And lifestyle changes can definitely have a big effect. A major clinical study that took place between 1998 and 2001—the Diabetes Prevention Program (DPP)—compared three groups of people who had been diagnosed with prediabetes. One group acted as a control group. Another group took the oral medication metformin. The third group received in-depth training encouraging weight loss through a healthy diet and exercise. The study found that the group who were taught to make lifestyle changes lowered their risk of developing full-blown diabetes by 58 percent! That was a better result than the group who received metformin, who lowered their risk by 31 percent. Never doubt that lifestyle changes can have a dramatic effect!

This book is one in a series that helps you explore the tools that you can use to manage your diabetes, especially the lifestyle changes you can make. This book focuses on the importance of exercise. We'll talk about things to consider as you get started with an exercise program, safety concerns you may have, and tips for sustaining an exercise program over time. As many people have discovered, it's not starting an exercise program that's the hardest part—it's sticking with it!

The book's biggest section consists of exercises you can try, accompanied by step-by-step instructions and photographs so that you can see and imitate proper form and posture. We've included an assortment of quick, easy aerobic and strength-training exercises that you can mix and match to build a perfect 10-minute workout. For those that suggest or require equipment such as weights or a fitness ball, you may want to borrow equipment from a friend or try the exercise out at a gym before you purchase any equipment, to see if these exercises are for you.

Keep in mind that you're not required to try out every exercise, or to stick with ones you don't enjoy—the goal is to find and use options that fit your fitness level. There isn't one single exercise program or type of exercise that you need to use. The most important thing is to get motivated, get up, and get moving!

GETTING STARTED

Regular exercise carries a lot of benefits for people with diabetes. It's a potent tool for lowering blood sugar because it improves the way insulin works. In fact, by incorporating regular exercise into their lives, many people with type 2 diabetes can increase their insulin sensitivity enough that they no longer need insulin injections or diabetes pills. For folks who have been diagnosed with prediabetes, it is even possible to prevent the full-blown disease through physical activity. The more calories the at-risk person burns per week by exercising, the lower their chances of progressing to type 2 diabetes!

Not only that, but physical activity is a proven way to combat conditions that often affect people with diabetes: heart disease, high blood pressure, infection, elevated cholesterol, depression, and increased stress. It burns extra calories—an important added benefit for those who need to lose weight. Physical activity also produces chemical messengers called endorphins that help relieve anxiety and pain.

In short, if you have diabetes, exercise is one of the most effective tools you can use to combat the disease. And if you're reading this book, you've probably made—or want to make—a commitment to an exercise program that will help you control your blood sugar and/or lose weight. But maybe you've been sedentary for a long time and need to find ways to get started. Maybe you've tried to include more exercise in your life before, but your plans have fizzled out after a few weeks. (Many people have had the experience of making a New Year's resolution that falters in the gray days of February and is forgotten by March!) Maybe you do exercise regularly, but you've recently received the diagnosis of diabetes and wonder if you need to make any changes based on your diagnosis. In the following pages, we'll discuss the factors you'll want to consider as you set up an exercise program. In later chapters, we'll talk about how exercise affects blood sugar and address potential health concerns, as well as suggesting some tips for maintaining your new routine.

STUDIES SAY

Sometimes it's difficult to block out time for exercise in your schedule. It can be easy to cancel a workout because the weather is bad or work is piling up—even to convince yourself that exercise doesn't really have that much of an effect. When you're having a hard time seeing the immediate benefits of exercise, remember that it definitely pays over the long-term. Researchers at the Cooper Institute in Dallas, Texas, rated the activity level of more than 1,200 men with type 2 diabetes. A dozen years later, they showed that men who were physically active on a regular basis and were moderately fit had a 60 percent lower death rate than unfit men who didn't exercise.

BEFORE YOU GET STARTED

We'll talk more about specific health concerns starting on page 25. Before you begin any exercise program, though, you'll want to talk to your primary care provider and other members of your diabetes care team. If you have certain complications caused by diabetes, you may be warned to steer clear of certain types of exercise. If you've been sedentary, your doctor or diabetes educator may have guidelines for how often or how intensely you should exercise in the beginning stages of your exercise program.

Your doctor or diabetes educator may also refer you to an exercise physiologist who can join your diabetes care team. (If they don't, and you are interested in the idea, ask for a referral.) An exercise physiologist can help tailor your fitness program to your goals and work with you as you meet those goals. When choosing an exercise physiologist, ask any potential candidates if they have experience working with people with diabetes. If you have any complications caused by diabetes, ask about their experience in working with people who have that condition. Verify that they have a degree or graduate-level training in exercise physiology; the American Diabetes Association notes that a certification from the American College of Sports Medicine is often a positive sign.

As with any member of your diabetes care team, you'll want to choose someone with whom you're comfortable. You'll be working together to devise an effective, challenging, and safe exercise program that evolves as your fitness increases. You'll want to be honest with this person, to feel that he or she listens to and addresses your concerns.

SETTING UP A SUSTAINABLE PROGRAM

Once you've gotten the go ahead from your diabetes care team, you'll want to think through what activities you'll include in your personal exercise program. The most important question when you're deciding whether an activity belongs in your program isn't how many calories it burns or how much it will lower your blood sugar. It's whether you'll do it. Set yourself up for success by incorporating things you enjoy—or, at a minimum, activities you don't dislike—in your exercise routine.

If you've been inactive for a while, this can be difficult. Sometimes you need to think outside the box, to activities you haven't thought of as exercise. Do you like to dance, but you only do so at weddings? If so, now's a great time to check out a social dancing class through your local park district or community center. Maybe you find the idea of a treadmill boring, but you like bird watching or admiring architecture—if you do, think about planning more nature hikes or walks through historic neighborhoods.

If you have a difficult time coming up with activities you might enjoy, think back to childhood. Was there a unit in gym that you liked more than the rest? See if a course for adults in that activity can be found through your local park district or community center. If you were a kid who liked climbing up trees, see if there's a gym with an indoor climbing wall in your area. Maybe you liked playing in the hotel pool when your family went on vacation—look into water aerobics classes through your local park district or a gym.

And don't be afraid to try something new. You might find that you enjoy the elliptical machine much more than the treadmill, or that you get a kick out of using a rowing machine. If you're competitive in other arenas, you might find that you can apply that competitive drive to games of tennis or racquetball.

BUILDING IN VARIETY

You've no doubt heard the aphorism that variety is the spice of life. It's also the key to a sustainable exercise program. You want to build a program with different types of exercise activities. That way, you won't only exercise the same muscles and joints. Having several potential activities to choose from can also keep you from getting bored and cutting your exercise time short.

Think about the weather—don't rely on activities that can only be performed in good weather. Even if you get a gym membership, incorporate some activities that you can do at home, so that you're not reliant on a working car to exercise.

If you travel a lot, look into things you can do on the road. Different types of exercise will also provide different health benefits. Some activities improve cardiovascular health. Some examples of good aerobic activities include cycling, walking, running, dancing, rowing, and swimming. These are all activities that engage large muscles in repetitive movement and raise your heart rate and breathing for an extended period of time.

Cardiovascular, or aerobic, exercise will tone your muscles, strengthen your heart, improve blood flow throughout your body, and help improve your blood sugar levels. But it won't necessarily do much to make your muscles bigger (if you're a man) or denser (if you're a woman). Adding muscle requires strength training, such as weight lifting. And strength training has its own health benefits. It helps turn fat into muscle, and that improves your basal metabolic rate.

Your basal metabolic rate refers to the calories your body burns just to keep your heart beating, lungs breathing, eyes blinking...in other words, just to keep you alive. This calorie expenditure is like the interest you earn on a bank account: It's essentially something you get for doing nothing but being there.

Fat is metabolically stagnant. In other words, fat cells require virtually no calories to stay alive. Muscle, on the other hand, is very active metabolically. Muscle cells chew through a lot of calories even when they aren't moving. The more muscle you have, the higher your basal metabolism and the more calories your body burns all the time—even when you're resting. Adding muscle is like turning a savings account that pays only 3 percent interest into a high-yield account that earns you 8 percent instead.

Strength training involves moderate to high exertion for short periods of time. When a muscle is worked to near (but not quite) exhaustion, the muscle becomes stronger and more efficient. Stronger and more efficient muscles burn more calories every minute of the day, whether you are actively working them or not, and they can help you achieve your weight loss goals more quickly.

STRENGTH-TRAINING TIPS

As with any form of exercise, when you start lifting

LOOKING FOR INSPIRATION?

Plenty of people with diabetes have competed in high-level sporting events. American swimmer Gary Hall, Jr., won ten medals (five gold, three silver, two bronze) in the 1996, 2000, and 2004 Olympic games. Sir Stephen Redgrave, a British rower, won six Olympic medals over the course of five different Olympic games. NFL quarterback Jay Cutler continued to play after he was diagnosed with type 1 diabetes in 2008. And legendary hockey Hall-of-Famer Bobby Clarke, who helped lead the Philadelphia Flyers to two Stanley Cup victories, played with diabetes throughout his professional career.

weights, it is best to start very slow and easy; otherwise, you could wind up very sore and discouraged afterward. As time goes on, gradually increase the number of repetitions (reps) you do of each weight-lifting exercise. Increase the amount of weight you use as well. Don't get discouraged if you reach a plateau and find it difficult to increase the weight or do additional reps; everyone hits plateaus at some points. Just work on perfecting your technique.

Here are some pointers to help make your weight-lifting workouts safer and more effective:

- Warm up before lifting. Walk or ride a stationary bike for a few minutes before you begin a round of weight lifting, and mimic each exercise (minus the weight) before performing it.

- Lift in the proper order. Start with exercises that work the big muscles in the chest, back, thighs, and shoulders, and end with lifts that train the smaller muscles of the arms and lower legs. When going through your lifting routine, try to alternate between exercises that work your arms and shoulders, those that strengthen your abdomen and lower back, and those that focus on your buttocks and legs.

- Never hold your breath when lifting weight. This can cause a dangerous rise in blood pressure. Blow air out when you raise the weight, and inhale as you lower it.

- Skip a day between weight-lifting workouts to give muscles time to recover and become stronger.

- When increasing weight, do so in very small increments. For example, go from lifting five pounds to six or seven pounds.

- Do not proceed until your technique is perfect. Be sure you can maintain the proper form for every single rep before you increase the weight or the number of reps. If you struggle with the last couple of reps, stay where you are until you can do them all properly.

- Lift and lower weight using slow, controlled movements. Slow lifts produce the best results.

LOW-IMPACT ACTIVITIES VS. HIGH-IMPACT ACTIVITIES

Another factor you'll want to consider is whether an activity is low-impact or high-impact. Low-impact activities are ones that don't involve a lot of jumping, pounding, or hitting anything with a lot of force, which can damage muscles, bones, and joints. If you haven't exercised regularly in some time, starting with low-impact activities can be a good idea. Swimming, cycling, hiking, and using an elliptical trainer all qualify as low-impact.

Those who have problems in their lower extremities would want to incorporate non-weight-bearing exercises such as stationary cycling, water exercise, and upper-body weight lifting. This includes anyone with very poor circulation or loss of nerve sensation in the legs or feet, as well as those with injuries, infections, or problems with balance.

If your fitness level allows, however, you can definitely enjoy higher-impact activities (such as running, jumping rope, boxing, or martial arts). If you have concerns, talk to your diabetes care team.

FREQUENCY AND DURATION

Exercise really does act like medicine for people with diabetes in that it changes the way the body uses insulin. While it's okay to take a day off every once in a while, it's best to get a daily dose of this medication. In fact, one study of people who successfully maintained long-term weight loss found that they had one important quality in common: They exercised for about one hour per day.

If you're new to exercise, start with just a few days per week. Increase the amount of exercise you do gradually, over time. Studies show that it takes at least 150 minutes of aerobic exercise per week to attain significant health benefits, including better blood sugar control, reduction of heart disease risk, and weight maintenance. The American Diabetes Association recommends spreading your weekly workout quota over at least three days, while not going more than two consecutive days without exercise. The ADA also recommends including strength training exercises twice a week.

If you can't fit in a long workout of 30 or 60 minutes, that's okay—break up your daily workout into 10-minute increments that you can fit into your day. The exercises we include in this book are examples of good short activities that you can squeeze into your day, or combine to form a longer workout.

SHOULD YOU JOIN A GYM?

When we think of exercise, one of the images that pop into our head is that of muscle-bound, healthy people working away at the gym. If you don't have a gym membership, you may have wondered if you should get one. Not necessarily. If you dread the very thought, your chances of using the membership decrease—and you don't want to set yourself up for failure or self-sabotage. (Along the same lines, it's not a great idea to invest a lot of money in creating a home gym full of equipment unless and until you're sure you will use with regularity.)

For some people, a gym might be the right choice. Some people like the availability of different equipment they can try, or the idea of having a specific place to go at a specific time. If you do want to join a gym, here are some factors to consider.

- What is the cost, and how are payments structured? How much notice do they give of price increases? Do you need to sign any contracts? How easy would it be to cancel the contract if, for example, you moved away? If you're using an introductory offer, how long does it last? What are the terms and price after the introductory offer expires? Does your membership renew automatically?

- How far away is the gym? Is it close to your workplace? Your home? Think about when you like to exercise, whether you're a morning person or a night owl—can you get to the gym easily and safely at that time?

- If they offer personal training sessions or classes, do they have anyone on staff who has worked with people with diabetes? What are the rates?

- When you talk to staff members about your fitness goals, do they listen, and do they respect those goals? Do they pressure you to join? If you ask for a tour, do they give you a thorough one?

- Can you get a free day pass? If so, go at the time you would usually want to go. How crowded is it? Do you have a long wait period for the machines you want to use? Are there any time limits on the popular machines? Are staff available to demonstrate how to use machines safely and effectively?

- What is the demographic of the people who use the gym? Some people feel self-conscious exercising around others, but better if those people fit in the same age bracket or fitness level.

- Is the equipment clean? Are the showers and the locker room clean and well-maintained?

- Is the gym a chain? If so, can you go to any gym in the chain or only one location?

Before you commit to anything, ask friends about their gyms, and if you can, look online for reviews.

Once you've decided what activities you're interested in, and where you'll exercise, you're ready to begin!

Measuring Intensity

How intensely should you exercise? Since your body is like no one else's, you'll need your own personal guide to tell you where to begin and how much physical effort you need to put in. Your best bet? Follow your heart. Your heart rate can tell you when you're working hard enough to increase your aerobic fitness.

Exercise physiologists have figured out a heart rate that is safe for most people during exercise. They call this your target heart-rate range. Your target heart-rate range is between 50 to 70 percent of your heart's maximal range (as measured by beats per minute). Your maximum heart rate is the number of times your heart beats when you're putting in your maximum effort.

This range tells you your optimum level of exertion during exercise. That doesn't mean you can't get any health or fitness benefits by exercising below or above that range. It's just that keeping your heart rate in the target heart-rate range during regular aerobic exercise has been shown to be safe and effective for increasing your aerobic fitness. In fact, exercising above this range can be very uncomfortable and may increase your risk of injury. If you've been inactive, however, it's best to start gradually. Exercise at a comfortable pace, one that may not get your heart rate in the target zone. Then gradually work your heart rate into the target zone.

So what is your target heart rate? The following table can act as a guide. Note that these ranges apply only to those who are not taking any medication that limits heart rate, such as beta blockers for high blood pressure; if you take any such medication, ask your doctor or exercise physiologist what your target range should be.

YOUR AGE	TEN-SECOND TARGET HEART-RATE RANGE DURING EXERCISE
20-29	20-26
30-39	19-25
40-49	18-23
50-59	17-22
60-69	16-21
70-79	15-19
80+	14-18

HOW AND WHEN TO MEASURE YOUR PULSE

To check your heart rate, you need a watch that measures seconds, not just minutes. You can take your pulse either at the radial artery in your wrist (on the inner side of your wrist, below the heel of your hand) or the carotid artery in your neck. Use the index and middle fingers of one hand to feel the pulse. If you use the artery in your neck, however, place your fingers gently; putting too much pressure on this artery can actually slow down your pulse and give you a false reading. When you've found your pulse, count the number of beats for ten seconds.

Check your pulse as you continue the activity, if possible; otherwise, stop only long enough to count the heartbeats. Counting your pulse for ten seconds will let you know if you are above, below, or within your target heart-rate range.

If your heart rate during exercise is above the range listed in the table on the previous page, slow down. If it is below, speed up a bit. Keep in mind that even if you maintain the same intensity, your heart rate may increase during the course of a workout as you begin to fatigue, so check your pulse every five or ten minutes throughout a longer workout to ensure you're still in your target range.

A word of caution: Don't be a slave to your pulse, measuring it so often that it becomes a compulsion. Don't let taking your pulse destroy your sense of fun and spontaneity in exercise.

As time goes on, you may only need to check your pulse at the beginning and end of your exercise workout; you may be able to tell whether you're working in your target range just by the way you feel.

RATING OF PERCEIVED EXERTION

As a matter of fact, one of the tools you can use to measure intensity, although a little less scientific, is nonetheless effective. It is called the Rating of Perceived Exertion scale, or RPE. Basically, you can use your perception of how hard you're working as a guide. If you really feel like you're working at a moderately intense pace, you probably are. Aim to keep your intensity in the "target zone" shown in the table below.

RPE ZONE	DESCRIPTION
0	Complete rest
1	Very, very easy
2	Very easy
3	Easy
4	**Moderately easy**
5	**Moderate**
6	**Moderately hard**
7	Hard
8	Very hard
9	Very, very hard
10	Absolute maximal effort

LISTEN TO YOUR BODY

There are three more principles that can guide you through your program. They should help you fight any tendency you may have to push yourself too hard—or to slack off.

First is the "talk test," which is especially important if you're returning to exercise after a period of being sedentary. The talk test means that you should be able to have a light, casual conversation while exercise. If you are too winded to talk, you can probably conclude that you're exercising too hard for your current fitness level. On the other hand, if you can sing, you probably need to push yourself harder.

Second, your exercise should be pain-free. If you experience a heaviness in your chest or any pain in your chest, jaw, neck, feet, legs, or back, you should slow down. If that doesn't stop the pain, see your doctor and describe what happened.

Third, if you seem excessively tired for an hour or more after exercise, your routine was too strenuous. Exercise should be exhilarating, not fatiguing. If you experience a dizzy or lightheaded feeling, it's time to back off. If you feel like vomiting or are tired the day after exercising, take it easy. If you can't sleep at night or if your nerves seem shot, it means you've been pushing too hard. The same is true if you seem to have lost your "zing" or can't catch your breath. These are your body's warning signs. If you have any questions about excessive fatigue, pain, or discomfort, see your doctor.

All three of these points stress listening to your body. It may take some practice, but you'll probably find it fun. You'll really get to know your body. And you'll learn that your body really can tell you when to speed up or slow down.

EXERCISING SAFELY

For people with diabetes, exercise can carry risk. To ensure that exercise doesn't cause more harm than good, read through and follow the guidelines below, and listen to any additional guidance given by your health care providers.

AVOID HYPOGLYCEMIA AND BLOOD SUGAR SPIKES

The more insulin you take—or the more insulin your body makes—the harder it is to burn fat and lose weight. But the opposite is also true: The less insulin you take (or make), the easier it is for your body to shed fat. That's why it's so important to take advantage of any opportunity that allows you to cut back on your insulin levels without harming blood sugar control.

Physical activity creates such an opportunity. Because physical activity makes your insulin work far more effectively, you don't need as much of it. In fact, if you inject insulin or use a medication that stimulates your pancreas to make more insulin, and you don't reduce your medication dose to account for physical activity, you could wind up with hypoglycemia.

If you do not use a medication that can cause hypoglycemia, you don't need to worry about snacking, reducing your medication dose, or doing anything else before or during your workouts to adjust for exercise. Medications that can cause hypoglycemia include insulin (all forms); sulfonylureas (glipizide, glyburide); meglitinides (Prandin, Starlix), and combination medications that contain any of the above.

If you do use insulin or a drug that increases your body's insulin production, you will need to make some common-sense adjustments that will help you prevent low blood sugar and lose weight faster. Just be sure to check with your diabetes care team before making any of your own dosage adjustments.

If you take rapid-acting insulin at mealtimes or use a pre-mixed formulation that contains rapid-acting insulin, it is a good idea to reduce your insulin dose at the meal prior to your physical activity. Work with your diabetes care team to determine doses that work for you.

Also, you should be prepared for the possibility of a delayed blood sugar drop, particularly after a long or very intense workout. There are two reasons such a drop can occur. The muscle cells' enhanced sensitivity to insulin, which normally occurs after activity, is prolonged when the exercise itself is prolonged. And the muscle cells need to replenish their own energy stores following such exhaustive exercise. If you tend to experience a drop in blood sugar several hours after heavy exercise, you can prevent it by lowering your long-acting and rapid-acting insulin by 25 percent following the workout or by having an extra snack prior to the time the drop in blood sugar tends to occur. Ideally, the snack should contain slowly digesting carbohydrates, such as whole fruit, milk, yogurt, or peanut butter.

If you take insulin or a medication that can cause hypoglycemia, there are certain situations in which you will need to consume extra food to prevent hypoglycemia. One example is when you will be exercising before or between meals. The size of the snack you'll need will depend on the duration and intensity of your workout. The harder and longer your muscles will be working, the more carbohydrate you will need to maintain your blood sugar level. The amount is also based on your body size: The bigger you are, the more fuel you will burn while exercising and the more carbohydrate you will need.

To confirm that you have chosen the optimal size and frequency for your snacks, test your blood sugar before and after the activity. If it has held steady, you chose the right amount. If it has gone up, you will need to cut back on the grams of carbohydrate you eat before each hour of exercise next time. And if your blood sugar has dropped, you will need to eat more carbohydrate before each hour of exercise or eat more frequently during your exercise session the next time.

If you take a medication other than insulin that can cause hypoglycemia, it is usually recommended that you take your usual dose for your first couple of exercise sessions and see what happens. If your blood sugar drops below 80 mg/dl during or after exercise, alert your diabetes care team. You may need to reduce or eliminate the medication or switch to a medication that does not cause hypoglycemia. Check with your doctor before you make any medication changes, however.

Despite the precautions you take, hypoglycemia can still occur if you take insulin or a medication that stimulates the release of insulin. So you should always carry a source of simple sugar (such as glucose tablets, a sports drink, juice, or hard candy) and wear a medical alert bracelet or necklace identifying you as a person with diabetes whenever you exercise. Stop the activity and treat the low blood sugar as soon as you suspect it, and take a timeout of at least 15 to 20 minutes to allow the food to be absorbed. Wait until your blood sugar is a minimum of 90 mg/dl before continuing physical activity.

Oddly enough, physical activity can actually increase blood sugar in certain circumstances, particularly at the onset of high-intensity, short-duration exercise. The cause is a surge of the stress hormone adrenaline. If you detect such an increase, talk with your doctor about ways to offset or prevent it. Although high blood sugar can impair your performance during exercise, it is not necessarily danger-ous to exercise when blood sugar levels are moderately elevated. If you experience high blood sugar during exercise, drink plenty of water during and after your workouts. If you experience very high blood sugar with exercise, alert your doctor and ask whether you should be checking your urine for ketones, which are acidic byproducts produced when fat is metabolized. It is a good idea to check for ketones if your blood sugar is greater than 300 mg/dl. A positive ketone test could mean that you are deficient in insulin, and in that case, physical activity will probably make your blood sugar go much higher. Do not exercise if you find your urine contains ketones.

By the numbers

- Avoid vigorous activity if your fasting glucose is above 250 mg/dl and you test positive for ketones.

- Exercise with caution if your fasting glucose is above 300 mg/dl in the absence of ketosis.

- Monitor blood sugar before, during, and after exercise. Comparing the results will provide important information about how exercise affects your insulin needs. Based on how your blood sugar changes after a workout, your doctor or diabetes educator will recommend necessary changes to your insulin dose and provide advice about whether you need to consume carbs before exercising. Since you will probably respond differently to a 30-minute swim than a 60-minute walk, be sure to do before-and-after testing for all the different activities you participate in.

- Consume carbs before exercising if your glucose level is below 100 mg/dl.

- Keep glucose tablets or another carb source handy in case you become hypoglycemic.

CHOOSING A TIME

Exercising at about the same time each day is best for improving blood sugar control and for sticking with an exercise program long-term. Because exercise can make your muscles more sensitive to insulin for several hours following the activity, exercising at the same time each day can help prevent unexpected peaks and valleys in your blood sugar levels. But if you need to vary the timing of your workouts because of other commitments, that's perfectly fine; just be prepared to make adjustments to your insulin or medication as needed.

If possible, you may want to take advantage of the immediate blood-sugar-lowering effect of exercise and do it soon after eating a meal. This especially benefits those who take insulin at each meal and want to lose weight, because they can cut back on their mealtime insulin dose and not have to worry about eating extra food just before exercising to ward off hypoglycemia. However, if you've been diagnosed with heart disease, it is best to wait a couple hours after a meal before exercising, as a weak heart may be overstressed when exercise is performed too soon after eating.

PROTECT YOUR FEET

Good-quality exercise equipment pays for itself in the form of better protection against injuries. In particular, good athletic shoes are a must for nearly all types of cardiovascular, or aerobic, exercise. Diabetes increases the risk of foot disease, and lower-limb diseases can progress quite quickly. When exercising, wear shoes with air or gel midsoles (the shock-absorbing pads between the soles and feet) and a generous toe box. Always wear socks to keep your feet dry.

Check your feet for blisters or cuts daily, especially if you engage in high-impact activities.

START SLOWLY AND COOL DOWN

When you exercise, include a few minutes of warm-up and cool-down time spent in a slow, easy version of your chosen exercise. If you plan to walk briskly for 30 minutes, for example, start and finish your workout with three to five minutes of casual walking before you increase your pace. This allows your heart rate to adjust gradually and safely as you begin and end your workout.

COMPLICATIONS

Although all diabetes patients should strive to be physically active, some forms of exercise require extra precautions (or may be too risky, period) for people who have any of the following complications.

Autonomic neuropathy. Patients who have this form of nerve damage may not be able to detect symptoms such as sweating and rapid heart rate that signal the onset of exercise-induced hypoglycemia. They also have a high risk for orthostatic hypotension (a drop in blood pressure that can cause dizziness or fainting) during exercise performed while upright, so cycling or swimming may be better choices than walking or running. Beware of exercising in very hot or cold climates, and drink plenty of water.

Diabetic retinopathy. Some types of physical activity increase the risk of a hemorrhage in the eye or a detached retina. Avoid activities that involve a lot of jarring or straining, such as jogging or weight lifting. Some yoga poses may also be off limits. Talk to your doctor or an exercise physiologist before engaging in yoga.

Peripheral neuropathy. If you can't feel your feet, how will you know if you're pounding the pavement too hard? People with serious loss of sensation in the lower limbs should not overdo weight-bearing exercise. Repetitive, intense pressure on the feet can cause ulcers. You may also fail to realize that you have broken a foot bone. If you have nerve damage that limits feeling in your feet, low-impact exercise, such as swimming, cycling, or rowing, may be the best choice.

DEALING WITH ACHES AND PAINS

No matter how carefully you exercise, you probably will experience a few little aches and pains—simply because you'll be asking your body to do things that it might not have done for years. Don't let a few minor physical discomforts discourage you. At the same time, don't persist in thinking that you should exercise until it hurts, or work through pain. Pay attention to your body.

MUSCLE SORENESS AND STIFFNESS

Even people who have been exercising regularly complain of occasional soreness and stiffness. The pain may occur immediately following the activity or after some delay, usually 24 to 48 hours. Often the discomfort lasts for only a few days. It is practically impossible to completely avoid muscle soreness and stiffness. But you can reduce the intensity of the pain by planning your conditioning program so that you progress gradually, especially during the early stages. That approach will allow the muscles of the body to adapt themselves to the stress placed on them. If you become sore and stiff from physical activity, doing some additional light exercises or general activity will often provide temporary relief.

MUSCLE CRAMPS AND SPASMS

When one of your muscles contracts powerfully and painfully, you may have a muscle cramp. The contraction may occur at any time—at rest as well as during activity. Cramps usually occur without warning. Occasionally, however, you may be able to feel one building up.

Among the causes of muscle cramps are fatigue; cold; imbalance of salt, potassium, and water levels; and over-stretching of unconditioned muscles. You can reduce the chances of muscle cramps by maintaining a proper diet, making sure you warm up properly prior to vigorous activity, and stopping activity before you become extremely fatigued.

If a cramp does occur, it can usually be stopped by stretching the muscle affected and firmly kneading it. Applying heat and massage to the area can restore circulation. If you're plagued with frequent cramps, drinking adequate fluid and eating foods with salt and potassium, along with muscle strengthening and stretching exercises, will usually eliminate the problem.

CHEST PAIN

Any chest pain, no matter what its cause, can be troubling—especially if you've reached middle age. Chest pain can be caused by factors that are in no way related to the condition of your heart. However, *chest pain should never be ignored or allowed to persist.* If you're ever in doubt about what's causing your chest pain, contact your health care provider.

Chest pain can be caused by **muscular causes**. A pulled pectoral (chest muscle) or a strained intercostal (side muscle) can cause a great deal of pain. A pulled muscle produces pain which is felt near the surface, and movements such as swinging the arm across the chest can initiate or worsen the pain. Bruised muscles and ligaments may cause pain during deep breathing, and they normally remain sensitive to the touch. Pain associated with this kind of condition usually only occurs during a certain motion and when pressure is applied to the area. Rest and time are usually the best treatments.

The pain brought on by indigestion, or **heartburn**, is frequently confused with heart pain, but it has nothing to do with the heart. Acid from the stomach backs up into the esophageal tube, causing contractions of the circular muscle of the esophagus. A simple diet of less highly seasoned food is the best prevention. Heartburn is often confused with real heart disease. If you can attribute the pain to a specific food, your worries are over. If you can't, see your doctor.

Angina pectoris usually develops during exercise, when emotion is high, or after a heavy meal. It is the result of a temporary failure of the coronary arteries to supply enough oxygenated blood to the heart muscle. Such a failure is usually caused by obstructions to coronary circulation.

Almost anyone can experience angina: people who have recovered from a heart attack, people who are going to have an attack, and some people who will never have an attack. The problem is that your heart muscle is simply not getting enough blood and oxygen. See your doctor if you suspect its presence.

Angina pain is usually not sharp; it usually is heavy, giving the victim the sensation that he or she is being squeezed or crushed in the center of the chest. The discomfort often spreads to the left shoulder, arm, or hand, where it may be felt as numbness. Pains may occur days, weeks, months, even years apart.

The pains associated with coronary heart disease are varied, yet similar to angina. They may be sharp or mild with a feeling of numbness. A good rule to follow regarding chest pain is that if the pain abruptly ends after exertion, see your physician.

If you experience any of these pains, particularly the kind that cause heavy pressure and radiate up the neck or down the arm, see your doctor. A very heavy pressure, as if someone were sitting on top of your chest; an extreme tightness, like a clenched fist inside the center of your chest; a feeling like indigestion, a stuffiness high in your stomach or low in your throat, may signal a heart attack. Whenever you have a strong symptom that resembles any one of these, stop exercising and get to your doctor.

STICKING WITH IT

For many people who have been sedentary, just getting motivated to start an exercise program can be a problem. Let's say you've overcome that hurdle. The next challenge is to stay motivated. Most people "attack" a fitness program, and after a few weeks, they quit. Your goal is to exercise on a regular basis and keep at it. Anybody can start an exercise program, but not everyone can stay at it.

Here are six ways to set yourself up for continued success.

1. **Set goals.** You're not going to get far without a specific objective. Goals are important. They give you something specific to work towards and a way to measure progress. When you're setting a goal, avoid vague generalizations: "I want to lose weight" or "I want to get into shape." Instead, set precise short-term, intermediate, and long-term goals. In the short-term, how many times can you commit yourself to exercising this week? In the intermediate term, over the next few months, is there a specific yoga pose you want to work on, a number of repetitions in your weight training you're working towards, or a number of miles you want to walk? In the long term, how many days a week do you want to exercise, and how much time will you spend each day? What are your goals in terms of blood sugar? Do you hope to maintain or cut down on the amount of medication you take?

Take stock of yourself right now. What would you like to do? What are you ultimately trying to achieve? Whatever it is, write it down. Even if it seems unrealistic at this time, put it in writing and save it. These are your long-term goals. Periodically, take out the sheet of paper and look at it. Write down your progress and what seems to be preventing you from achieving your goals.

Plan how you are going to reach your goals. Write it down, and be specific. If you're working towards spending thirty minutes a day in exercise and you're only spending five, can you increase by one minute a day? Jot down some motivators.

If you're having trouble with your intermediate or long-term goals, start small. What can you do today?

2. **Record your progress.** For some people, what makes watching a sport really interesting is competition. If that's true for you, look for ways to compete with yourself. Just use a progress log (see page 127 for a sample exercise log that you can use as a jumping off point). A log lets you compete with yourself. It tells you and anyone else who looks at it how well you're doing and how close you're getting to your goal. It gives you a sense of accomplishment. It helps you form future goals.

3. **Make a time commitment.** Have you ever noticed how easily you slip into routines? Perhaps you always brush your teeth before, not after, you shower in the morning; always

put your left, not your right, shoe on first; take the same route to work every day. And have you ever noticed how you tend to feel you've forgotten to do something important if anything should interfere with this little ritual? You may find it easier to stick with an exercise program if you can allow it to become part of your daily routine—so much a part that you'll feel compelled to exercise despite your own excuses for skipping a day. If you can get yourself into the habit of exercising at a certain time every day, you'll accept it as part of your regular daily schedule and not just something to do during odd moments.

4. **Choose the best time of day.** The best time depends on you. Listen to your biological clock. Don't try to force yourself into a mold. If you're a lark, exercise in the morning. If you're not, don't try to wedge it into your day then—you don't want to have to fight the temptation to hit "snooze" on the alarm clock every day. If you're an owl, exercise in the evening—though you'll want to keep an eye on your night-time blood sugar levels to make sure you're not headed for a hypoglycemic episode during the night. If the afternoon if your time of day, do it then. Whatever time is appropriate, make sure to give yourself a time commitment. You must be willing to set aside a certain period of time each day or every other day.

At first a little experimenting may be necessary to find out what works best for you. You'll also want to keep an eye on your food intake and the interaction of your blood sugar with any medication/insulin you take.

5. **Put yourself in a positive frame of mind.** What happens in your head is almost as important as what happens to your body, because if you don't enjoy what you're doing, you'll begin to find reasons for not doing it.

Before you exercise, try to get yourself into a positive, active frame of mind. As you exercise, be aware of what's happening to your body. Feel your muscles work. Concentrate on the rhythmic flow of your movements.

6. **Enlist a workout pal.** If you have a spouse or partner, encourage them to work out with you, or seek out a friend. Working out with a friend gives you the advantage of companionship and encouragement—and maybe a bit of healthy competition! Sometimes, when you would skip a day yourself, you won't if it would mean cancelling on a friend.

Walking for Health

Walking is so simple that we often overlook it as a form of exercise. But it has a lot of advantages. You don't need fancy gear or equipment. It's low impact. And you can fit a brisk 10-minute (or longer) walk into your way of life more easily than almost any other kind of exercise. It burns calories, too—in general, a 150-pound person walking at average speed (from two to three-and-a-half miles per hour) will burn about 80 calories a mile.

Although not as strenuous as jogging, walking will increase your heart rate and oxygen consumption enough to qualify as an aerobic exercise. When you walk, your heart starts to beat faster and move larger amounts of oxygen-rich blood around your body more forcefully. Your blood vessels expand to carry this oxygen. In your working muscles, unused blood vessels open up to permit a good pickup of oxygen and release of carbon dioxide. These changes improve your ability to process oxygen. And better circulation to your leg muscles can mean less leg fatigue and fewer aches.

The aerobic benefits aren't the only ones you'll get by incorporating walking into your life. Walking can refocus your attention from whatever is troubling you, reducing anxiety, tension, and stress. It helps you relax and recharge your mind and body. In the pages that follow, we'll discuss some tips for getting the most out of a walking routine.

YOUR POSTURE AND STRIDE

Walk naturally. Your body is unique. It has its own construction and balance, so you can't force it to behave exactly like someone else's. It is good to keep your spine straight and hold your head high as you walk, but try not to be so conscious of this that you feel unnatural.

Don't exaggerate your arm motions. Allow your arms to hang loosely by your sides. They will swing in the opposite action of your legs. Keep your hands, hips, knees, and ankles relaxed. As you walk, don't worry about the length of your stride. Just do whatever is comfortable.

Each foot should strike the ground at your heel. The weight is then transferred from your heel up along the outer border your foot towards your toes. Then you should push off with your toes to complete the foot strike pattern. As you move from heel to toe, you will get a rolling motion. Avoid landing flat-footed and on the balls of your feet.

Don't follow these guidelines slavishly. It's likely that the way you walk already is best for you. Remember, you're walking for fitness and fun. Don't worry about style or form.

PROTECT YOUR FEET

The most important equipment you can own when walking is your shoes. You can cover just as much territory in old cut-off shorts and a T-shirts as you can in an expensive outfit. But a good pair of shoes spells the difference between pain and comfort, success and failure.

Each mile you walk, your foot hits the ground about 400 times. Good shoes are essential to protecting your feet and avoiding injuries. Look for running shoes that give good support. Why running shoes for walking? Because they provide the support, protection, comfort, and cushioning that your feet will need for walking on all kinds of surfaces. When you try on a new pair of shoes, be sure they fit well in the toe.

Always wear socks that are clean and fit snugly. Wear a material that will absorb moisture well.

Socks and shoes aren't the only factor in protecting your feet. When you choose a route, pay close attention to the surfaces you're walking on. A lot of walkers say grass or packed dirt is the best surface for walking. These surfaces are soft, so they are good for shock absorption. Ideally, the surface is also smooth enough to allow you to walk quickly without tripping. If the grass or dirt is too clumpy, it won't provide good enough traction and you may stumble or fall.

If you can't find a nice, springy green surface to use, pavement is an alternative. But it does have its drawbacks. Some foot and leg problems are either caused or aggravated by walking on hard surfaces like concrete or asphalt. Watch for uneven surfaces and potholes, and avoid congested areas where there is a lot of stop-and-go traffic. Remember also that asphalt tends to absorb more heat than concrete, so it can make your feet hotter during warm-weather walks.

Walking indoors is also an option. If you walk on an indoor track, it is best to switch directions every other day. By walking counterclockwise one day and clockwise the next, you will help avoid orthopedic problems that can result from walking on a surface that slopes to the left or right. You can also try out a treadmill. (Don't buy a treadmill unless you've tried one out and know you'll use it, though! If you do decide to purchase one, it's a good idea to try it out in the store.)

DISTANCE AND SPEED

HELPFUL GEAR

If you're walking on hilly terrain or have any concerns about your balance or stability, consider a pair of walking/ trekking poles. If you do, make sure you adjust them for your height and stride.

As with any exercise program, don't let your enthusiasm trick you into overdoing it. You don't want to set a pace that you can't maintain, because you will just become exhausted and discouraged, and you'll increase your risk of injury. Don't plan for a 10-mile hike on your first day. Instead, try to fit three 10-minute walks into your day. Maybe you walk on a treadmill in the morning, take a walk around the block during your lunch break, and invite your spouse or partner to take a walk with you after dinner.

As for pace, don't worry about speed. One easy rule is to follow the talk test. When walking, breathe naturally. If you feel comfortable with your mouth closed, close it. If not, then open it. Remember, the faster you go, the more air you'll need. Note that you should be able to hold a conversation with someone beside you as you go. Even when you walk alone, you can use your imagination: do you feel like talking? If not, you're probably walking too fast for your present fitness level.

HILLS AND STAIRS

Walking up hills and stairs burns extra calories and raises your heart rate more than walking at the same speed on a flat surface. Thus, it does an even better job of helping you to control your weight and build your aerobic capacity. It also provides more of a workout for the large muscles in the buttocks and the muscles in the front of the thighs, which are responsible for lifting the legs, climbing, and pushing off.

HOW FAR CAN YOU GO?

Keep track of how far you walk! Pedometers can be found at most department stores and sporting goods stores. You don't need one that's fancy or complicated. All you need it to do is count your steps. As long as it has a button that lets you reset it each day, it should suit your needs.

With the heightened benefits, however, comes an increase in your risk of injury. Some simple adjustments in your walking technique can help you hold down your risk. While walking uphill, walk slightly slower and lean forward. Downhill walking is harder on the bones and joints; to minimize the shock of the downhill landing forces, shorten the length of your stride.

FIT WALKING INTO YOUR DAY

Don't just add walking to your day—if sidewalks and safety permit, replace some of your daily driving time with walking. Do you have any grocery stores within a half-mile or mile radius? If so, invest in a push cart and walk there and back. You can also incorporate walking into your daily commute. Maybe the total distance to work is too long to walk. However, instead of getting off at the bus stop closest to work, can you get off one or two stops earlier? If you take the train in to work, can you walk to the train in the morning or leave your car at a parking lot that's further out? If you didn't pack a lunch, instead of hopping into a car at lunchtime, can you walk to any nearby restaurants?

If you are walking along public roads at any point, follow basic safety guidelines. Wear light-colored clothes, and consider wearing some kind of reflective tape, too. If you are walking at dawn, dusk, or in the evening, carry a flashlight so you can see where you are walking and so you can alert motorists to your presence.

Always know the road you are walking on so that you'll know where curves, ditches, and uneven pavement loom.

WHATEVER THE WEATHER?

Some days, the weather is ideal for walking: very light breeze, temperature around 60 degrees, no clouds in sight. But what do you do when the snow starts to fall or the heat makes you feel as though your shoes will melt? It may not sound appealing, but you can walk in most weather conditions. If you succeed in making a walking program as much a part of your day as eating or sleeping, you'll probably find yourself walking through rain, snow, and sleet—and even enjoying it. However, temperature extremes can be more than uncomfortable; they can be dangerous if you do not prepare yourself adequately.

If you have a heart condition, ask your doctor if it is all right for you to brave very cold weather. High wind-chill factors are the greatest threat in cold weather, since you can get frostbite if you are inadequately protected from the wind. Be sure that all normally exposed areas of your skin—head, face, ears, and hands—are covered. Dress in layers of clothing that will keep the heat in and the cold out. In cooler weather, it's generally better to wear layers that you can take off than to be cold from the start.

When it is hot, be especially careful. You don't want to walk yourself into heat exhaustion. Drink water before, during, and after your walk. Wear light clothing that absorbs sweat and allows it to evaporate easily. Wear sunscreen. Some people like to wear a lightweight cap that will reflect the sun's rays. After the thermometer hits a certain temperature, though, don't try to walk, especially if it's humid.

KEEPING UP YOUR INTEREST LEVEL

You may find yourself walking for longer distances and longer periods of time. That's great! If you're doing so, here are some recommendations for maintaining your interest level over time.

1. Vary your route and your scenery. Research trails at local parks and forest preserves. Look into memberships at arboretums or botanical gardens. If you live near a historic neighborhood or cemetery, see if a local historical society puts out a do-it-yourself walking tour. While making discoveries, always consider safety and take traffic into account. Check over the route you plan to use ahead of time.

2. Find a buddy. This can be a little tricky, as you want to find someone who is compatible in terms of pace, goals, and the amount of conversation you'll have—you don't want to find yourself slowing down to an amble while you chat away, but neither do you want to huff and puff to keep up with someone who speeds along. But if you can find someone, it's a great way to stay accountable and interested. You might even look into a local hiking group (check meetup.com).

3. Walk to music, a podcast, or an audio book. If you do have earbuds in, though, take care that you are remaining aware of your surroundings in other ways.

4. Record your mileage on a map. Your regular walking route may take you around the same section of your neighborhood each day, but you can mark off your distance on a map as though you were walking cross-country. You can even set yourself up for a reward that way—if you walk the distance equivalent to a nearby city, reward yourself with a day trip there!

CARDIO EXERCISES

GUIDELINES FOR USING THE ELLIPTICAL

Elliptical trainers are a great source of cardiovascular training. They are a high intensity, low-impact machine that causes less stress on the joints than treadmills or jogging. There are two types of ellipticals: ones with stationary arms and ones with moveable arms. The type with moveable arms will get the upper body moving, adding a greater calorie burn. People with balance issues should use caution when getting on and off the machine, as the pedals are not stationary. Because ellipticals are weight-bearing exercise, people with neuropathy of the feet should be cautious when using these machines and, if possible, use a recumbent elliptical to take pressure off the feet.

The cardio goal for exercisers with diabetes is to reach 30 minutes of aerobic exercise, five days a week. For beginners this may not be possible. Try doing smaller increments, for example, 5–10 minutes, multiple times per day.

Once the 30 minutes has been achieved, try changing the workout by adding intervals, hills, or one of the other programmed workouts. Letting go of the handles can also change the intensity of the workout by adding a balance challenge and strengthening the core muscles.

MARCH IN PLACE

Marching in place is a low-intensity, moderate-impact exercise. Like other cardio activities, it increases the heart rate to strengthen the heart and lungs while also increasing circulation throughout the body. If neuropathy of the feet is present, do seated.

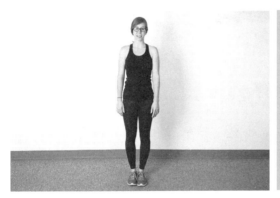

STEP 1
Stand (or sit) tall with abdominals pulled in.

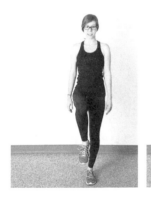 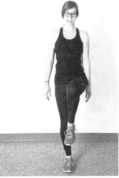

STEP 2
March in place for 1–2 minutes.

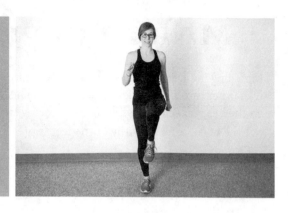

RUN IN PLACE

Running in place is a moderate-intensity, moderate-impact exercise. Avoid this exercise if neuropathy of the feet is present.

STEP 1
Stand tall with abdominals pulled in.

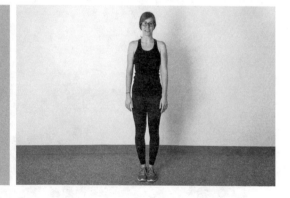

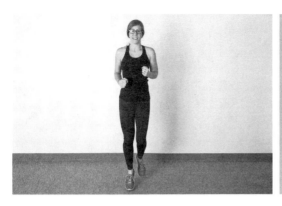

STEP 2
Run in place for
1–2 minutes.

STEP 3
For added
intensity,
swing arms.

HEEL TAPS

Heel taps are a low-intensity, low-impact exercise. Along with
providing cardiovascular benefits, heel taps also aid in stretching
the back of legs and ankles.

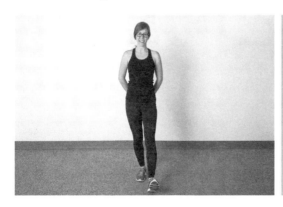

STEP 1
Stand (or sit) tall
with abdominals
pulled in. Using
a quick pace,
alternating legs,
tap heels on floor
for 1–2 minutes.

STEP 2
As you do this exercise, keep toe pointed to ceiling.

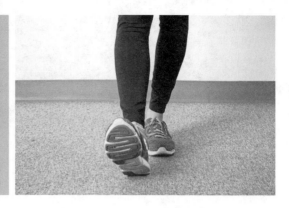

STEP 3
For added intensity, add an arm reach to ceiling.

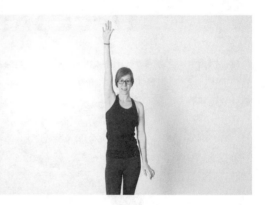

TOE TAPS

Toe taps are a low-intensity, low-impact exercise. Along with providing cardiovascular benefits, toe taps also aid in stretching the front of legs and ankles.

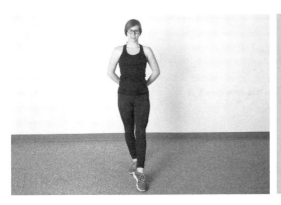

STEP 1
Stand (or sit) tall with abdominals pulled in. Using a quick pace and alternating legs, tap toes on floor for 1–2 minutes.

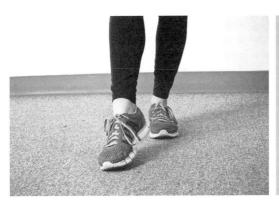

STEP 2
As you do this exercise, keep toe pointed to floor.

STEP 3
For added intensity, add an arm reach to ceiling.

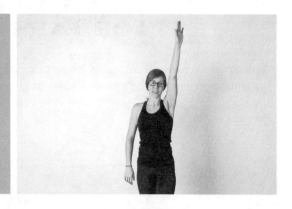

JUMP ROPE

Jumping rope is a moderate-intensity, high-impact exercise. Jumping rope can be done with a rope or by twirling the arms without a rope. If neuropathy of the feet is present, do this exercise in a chair, omitting the rope.

STEP 1
Stand (or sit) tall with abdominals pulled in. Begin to hop in place, twirling arms forward or using a jump rope. Hop for 1–2 minutes.

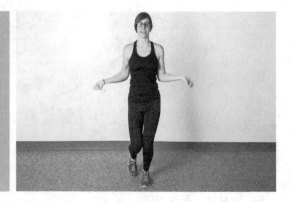

HIGH KNEES

High knees are a moderate-intensity, moderate-impact exercise. Along with providing cardiovascular benefits, high knees also aids in strengthening the hip and core muscles. If neuropathy of the feet is present, do seated.

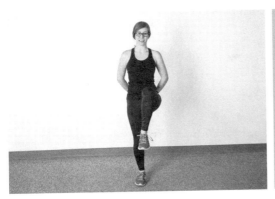

STEP 1
Stand (or sit) tall with abdominals pulled in. Alternating legs, pull knees to hip level.

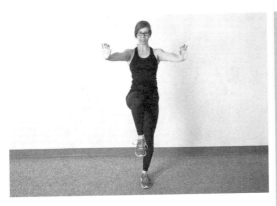

STEP 2
As you do this exercise, keep spine straight. Lift knees for 1–2 minutes.

STEP 3
For added intensity, add a forward press with arms.

SIDE STEPS

Side steps are a low-intensity, moderate-impact exercise. Along with providing cardiovascular benefits, side steps strengthen the outer and inner thighs. If neuropathy of the feet is present, do seated.

STEP 1
Stand (or sit) tall with abdominals pulled in. Step both feet to the left and then step both feet to the right.

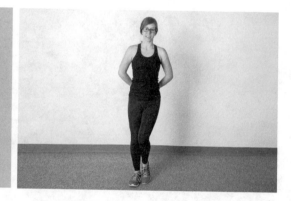

STEP 2
Step side to side for 1–2 minutes. For added intensity, add pulling movement with arms.

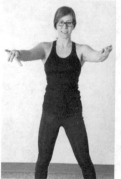
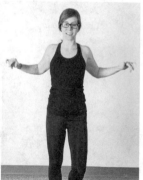

FORWARD AND BACK STEP

Stepping forward and back is a low-intensity, moderate-impact exercise. Along with providing cardiovascular benefits, stepping forward and back aids in training the walking and balance muscles of the upper leg. If neuropathy of the feet is present, do seated.

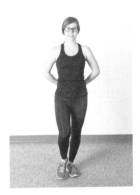 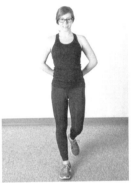

STEP 1
Stand (or sit) tall with abdominals pulled in. Step both feet forward.

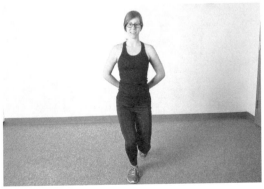

STEP 2
Step both feet back. Step forward and back for 1–2 minutes.

STEP 3
For added intensity, add a knee bend with the forward step.

JUMPING JACKS

Jumping jacks are a high-intensity, high-impact exercise. If neuropathy of the feet is present, modify exercise or do seated.

STEP 1
Sit (or stand) tall, abdominals pulled in. Jump feet out to either side while bringing arms up overhead. Then return to start. Jump for 1–2 minutes.

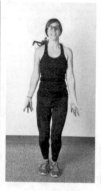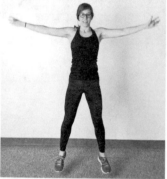

STEP 2
To modify, alternate side taps with feet while bringing arms up over head.

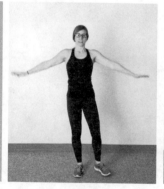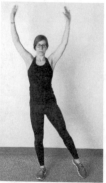

STRENGTH EXERCISES

All strength exercises should be done with weights or resistance tubing that challenges the muscles. Suggested resistance would be 5–10 lb hand weights or light to moderate resistance tubing. For leg exercises, light ankle weights or circular resistance bands are beneficial for strengthening the lower body muscles.

BICEP CURLS

Bicep curls are a low-intensity, no-impact exercise. This exercise strengthens the front of the arm, the muscle used for lifting and rotating the arm outward.

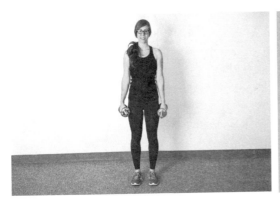

STEP 1
Stand (or sit) tall, feet at hip distance.

STEP 2

Put arms straight down by sides, palms turned in toward body.

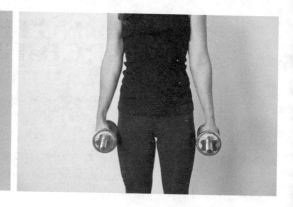

STEP 3

Keeping the elbows close to ribs, curl hands up towards shoulder. Rotate palms to ceiling.

STEP 4

The exercise can be done with one or both arms. Do 10–15 repetitions.

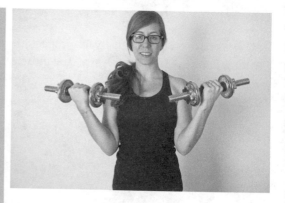

LATERAL RAISE

Lateral raises are a low-intensity, no-impact exercise. This exercise strengthens the shoulder muscles that are used for lifting and rotating the arms.

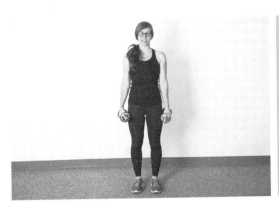

STEP 1
Stand (or sit) tall, feet at hip distance. Put arms straight down by sides, palms turned in toward body.

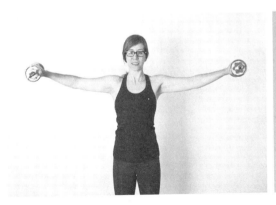

STEP 2
Lift one or both arms out to side, elbows slightly bent. Do not lift higher than the shoulder joint. Do 10–15 repetitions.

CHEST PRESS

This exercise is a low-intensity, no-impact exercise. The chest press will strengthen the chest muscles, which are important for pushing movements. This group of muscles also aids in maintaining good posture.

STEP 1
Stand (or sit) tall, feet at hip distance. Hands should be at chest height, palms facing down, elbows out.

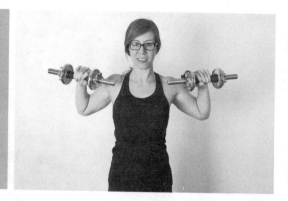

STEP 2
Press arms forward. Do not lock elbows.

STEP 3
Return to start position. Do 10–15 repetitions.

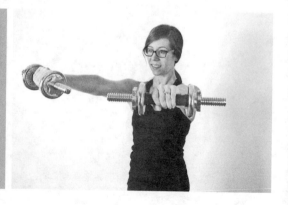

PRESS BACK

The press back exercise is a low-intensity, no-impact exercise. This exercise strengthens the upper back muscles, which are important for pulling movements. This group of muscles also aids in maintaining good posture.

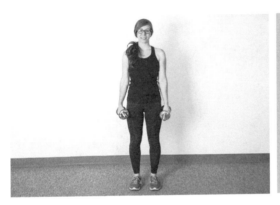

STEP 1
Stand (or sit) tall, feet at hip distance. Arms should be straight down by sides.

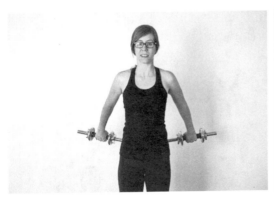

STEP 2
Face palms backward. Lift one or both arms back, squeezing shoulder blades. Keep shoulders relaxed. Do 10–15 repetitions.

SIDE LEANS

This exercise is a low-intensity, no-impact exercise. Side leans strengthen the muscles at the sides of the waist, which are part of the "core" muscle group. The core muscles aid in posture maintenance, bending, and twisting the midsection of the body. This group of muscles also contributes to posture maintenance and improving balance.

STEP 1

Stand (or sit) tall, abdominals pulled in. Arms should be straight down by sides, with the spine as straight as possible.

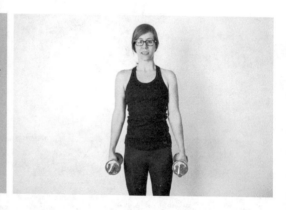

STEP 2

Keeping the spine long, lean to the left, crunching side of waist.

STEP 3

Do 10–15 repetitions. Repeat on other side.

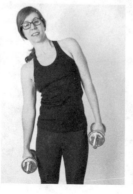
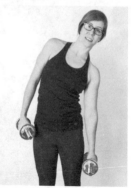

CRUNCHES

Crunches are a low-intensity, no-impact exercise. This exercise strengthens the front of the abdominals, which are part of the "core" muscle group. The front of the abdominals are the muscles responsible for bending forward; they also aid in posture maintenance and improving balance. Be cautious of this exercise if osteoporosis of the spine is present. This exercise can be done seated or laying on the floor.

IN CHAIR

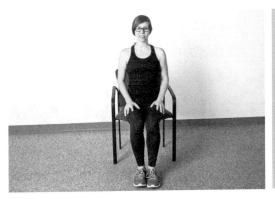

STEP 1
Sit tall with abdominals pulled in.

STEP 2

Cross arms in front of chest.

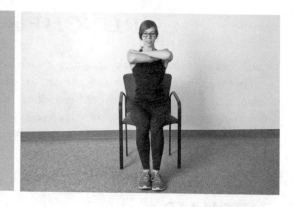

STEP 3

Keeping abdominals tight, bend forward to tap elbows to knees. Keep lower back pressing into chair. Do 10–15 repetitions.

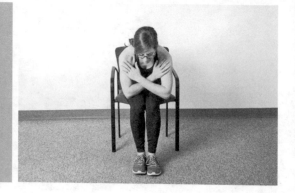

LYING ON FLOOR

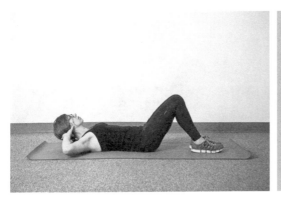

STEP 1
Lie on floor, knees bent, feet flat. Place hands behind head for neck support.

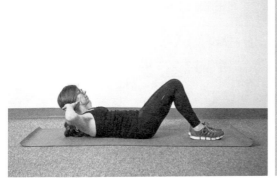

STEP 2
Keeping abdominals tight, press lower back into floor, curling head and shoulders up.

STEP 3
Do not pull on neck. Do not lift your lower back off floor.

STEP 4
Return to start position. Do 10–15 repetitions.

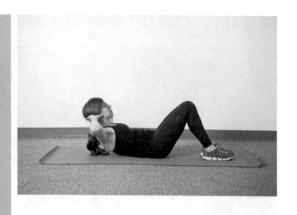

DEAD LIFT

This is a moderate-intensity, no-impact exercise. Dead lifts strengthen the muscles that run along the spine, which are important for posture maintenance and balance. Even though these muscles are located on the back, they are still an important part of the "core" muscle group. Be cautious of this exercise if lower back pain or spinal stenosis is present.

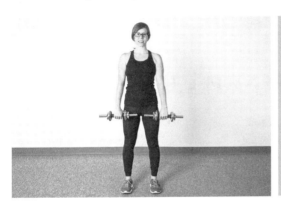

STEP 1
Stand (or sit) tall, abdominals pulled in. Arms should be hanging straight down by sides, palms facing backward.

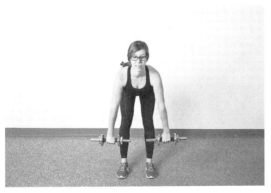

STEP 2
Keeping arms straight, bend forward with straight spine until body is at 90 degree angle.

STEP 3

Press weight down through heels (hips, if seated). Slowly lift upper body back to start position. Do 10–15 repetitions.

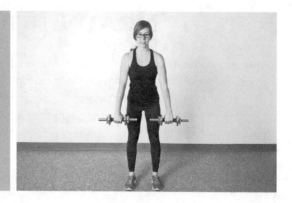

KNEE LIFT

Knee lifts are a low-intensity, low-impact exercise. This exercise strengthens the hip muscles. Be cautious of this exercise if hip pain or injury is present. An ankle weight can be used.

STEP 1

Stand (or sit) tall. Lift bent left knee to hip height.

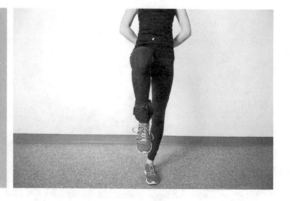

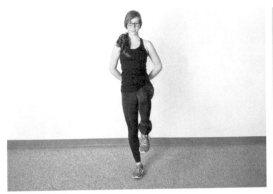

STEP 2
Keep foot flexed.
Do 10–15
repetitions.

STEP 3
Repeat with
other leg.

FORWARD KICK

This exercise is a low-intensity, low-impact exercise. Forward kicks strengthen the thigh muscle. Be cautious of this exercise if knee pain or injury is present. An ankle weight can be used.

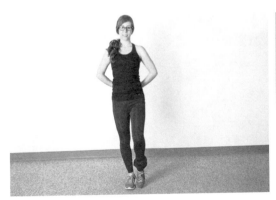

STEP 1
Stand (or sit) tall.
Slightly bend
knee, placing toe
of left foot on
floor. If seated,
begin with knees
bent, feet flat.

STEP 2

Straighten leg; focus on squeezing thigh. Do 10–15 repetitions.

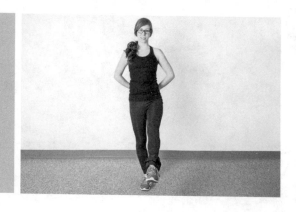

STEP 3

Repeat with other leg.

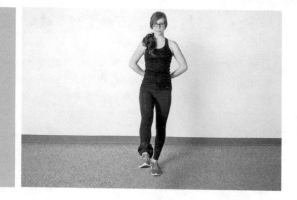

LEG CURL

The leg curl exercise is a low-intensity, no-impact exercise. This exercise strengthens the muscles at the back of the thigh, which are important for bending the knee and walking. Be cautious if knee pain or injury is present. An ankle weight can be used.

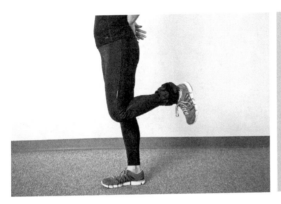

STEP 1
Stand tall, feet at hip distance. With left foot flexed, bend left knee, bringing foot backward.

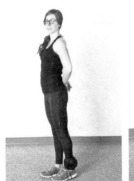 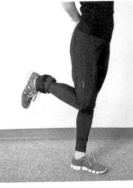

STEP 2
Keep knees close together. Lower to start position. Do 10–15 repetitions. Repeat with other leg.

SIDE LEG RAISE

This exercise is a low-intensity, no-impact exercise. Side raises strengthen the inner and outer thigh muscles, which are important for side to side movements. Be caution of this exercise if hip pain or injury is present.

STEP 1
Stand tall, feet at hip distance. Keeping upper body tall, lift straight leg to the side. Keep foot relaxed.

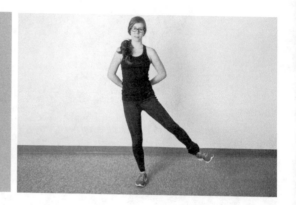

STEP 2
Return to start position. Do 10–15 repetitions.

STEP 3
Repeat with other leg.

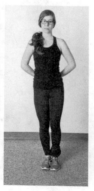
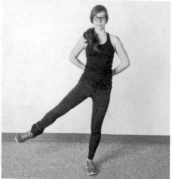

Heel Raises

Heel raises are a low-intensity, low-impact exercise. This exercise strengthens the calf muscles. If neuropathy of the foot is present, do this exercise seated.

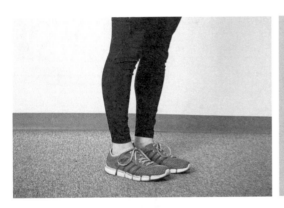

STEP 1
Stand (or sit) tall, feet at hip distance.

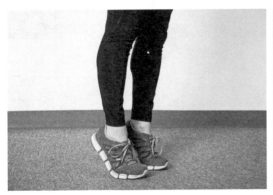

STEP 2
Keeping upper body tall and legs straight (knees bent, if seated), lift one or both heels off the ground. Do 10–15 repetitions.

SQUATS

Squats are a moderate-intensity, no-impact exercise. Squats challenge all of the muscles of the upper leg, which are important for the fundamental movements of our lower body, such as walking, bending the knees, lifting the legs, and getting in and out of a chair. If hip or knee problems are present, do partial squats or avoid this exercise.

STEP 1
Stand with feet at hip distance. Pull in abdominals to protect lower back.

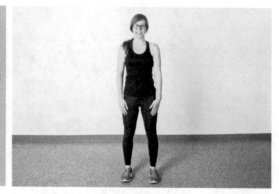

STEP 2
Bend knees and move hips back, as if sitting in a chair. Do not take knees further forward than toes.

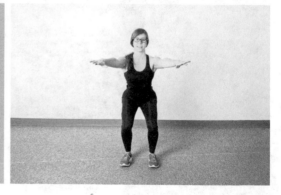

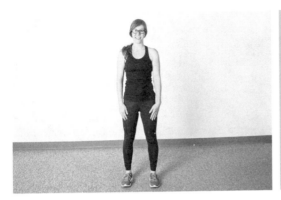

STEP 3
Press weight through heels to return to standing position. Do 10–15 repetitions.

LUNGES

Lunges are a moderate-intensity, no-impact exercise. This exercise strengthens the muscles of the thigh. If knee pain or injury is present, avoid this exercise.

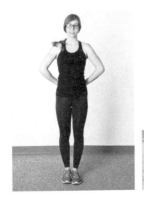 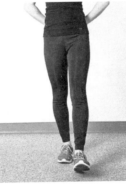

STEP 1
Stand tall with feet at hip distance. Step left foot forward into staggered stance.

STEP 2
Keeping upper body tall, bend both knees to 90 degrees. Do not let knees go past the toes.

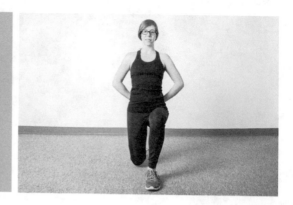

STEP 3
Return to standing position. Do 10–15 repetitions.

STEP 4
Repeat with other leg.

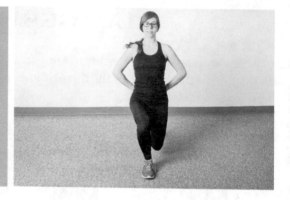

FITNESS BALL
PELVIC CIRCLES

This exercise is designed to enhance core strength and improve balance. Pelvic circles are low intensity and add no impact to the spine. This exercise is a challenge for those with balance issues, so use the ball with caution.

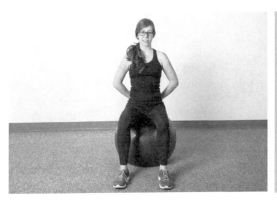

STEP 1
Sit on a stability ball with feet flat on the floor, spine tall. Pull the abdominals in toward the spine.

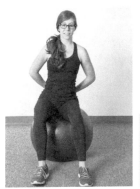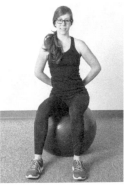

STEP 2
Make a circular motion with the hips moving in a clockwise direction. Do 15 repetitions, then repeat going the other direction.

HIP EXTENSIONS

Hip extensions target the hips and legs, both important muscles for walking. Adding the stability ball engages the core muscles and adds a balance challenge to the exercise. This is a no-impact, moderate-intensity exercise.

STEP 1
Lie flat on your back with ankles resting on a stability ball, legs straight.

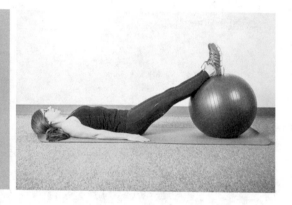

STEP 2
Keeping legs straight and abdominals contracted, lift hips towards ceiling. Keep neck and shoulders relaxed.

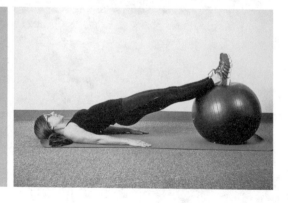

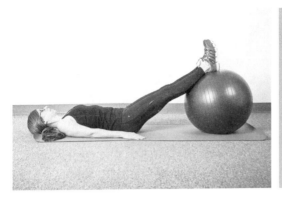

BACK EXTENSIONS

This exercise is a low-intensity back exercise that helps to improve posture and core strength. Back extensions are of moderate impact to the spine, so people with spinal stenosis should avoid this exercise.

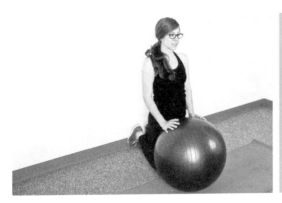

STEP 1
Bring the ball to an area with a wall nearby. Kneel in front of the ball. Lean forward, placing abdominals on the ball.

STEP 2

Straighten legs, securing feet against a wall.

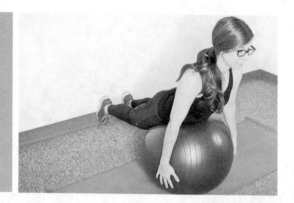

STEP 3

Round the upper body forward so it is draped over the ball.

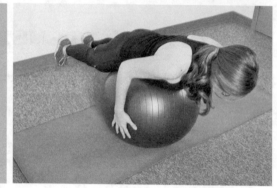

STEP 4

Lift the head and shoulders up until upper body is in line with lower body. Do not extend beyond a straight spine. Do 10–15 repetitions.

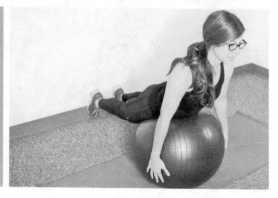

WALL SQUAT

Wall squats are a moderate-intensity, moderate-impact exercise designed to strengthen the legs. This exercise also engages the core muscles. If knee pain is present, only squat halfway or to tolerance. Use caution if suffering from peripheral neuropathy.

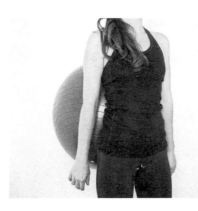

STEP 1
Stand with back to wall, ball resting against lower back. Feet should be hip distance apart.

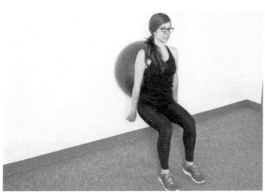

STEP 1
Keeping upper body straight and abdominals contracted, lower the hips and bend the knees. Be sure that knees are not going past toes.

STEP 3
Press weight
down through
the heels to press
back up to
standing.

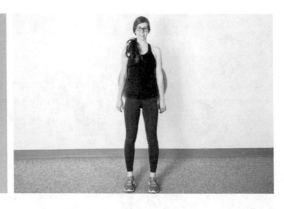

PLANK

This is a high-intensity, no-impact exercise. It is a whole-body
strength builder and an excellent balance training exercise. Plank
can be done either in a modified, kneeling position or in full,
straight leg position.

STEP 1
Kneel on the
floor in front of
a stability ball.

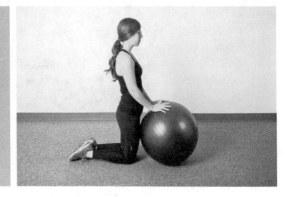

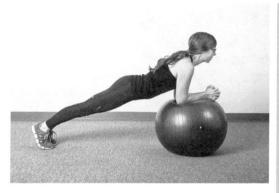

STEP 2

Placing elbows on ball, shift weight forward onto elbows. Keep abdominals engaged and hold for 3 deep breaths. Stay in this position for modified plank.

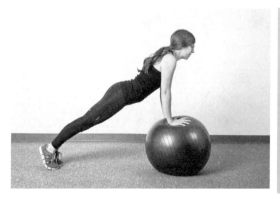

STEP 3

Move into full plank by straightening arms. Maintain straight line between shoulders and ankles. Do not let hips drop. Hold for 3 deep breaths.

PUSH UP

Ball push ups are a high-intensity exercise that strengthens the upper back and chest. The addition of the ball engages the core muscle and aids in balance training. This exercise can be done in a modified kneeling position or in full, straight leg position.

STEP 1

Kneel on floor in front of stability ball. Place hands shoulder distance apart, palms flat against the ball.

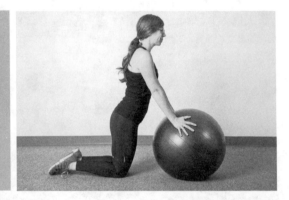

STEP 2

For modified push ups, remain on knees. Lower upper body towards the ball, pause, push back up to start position. Keep chin up and abdominals engaged. Do 10–15 repetitions.

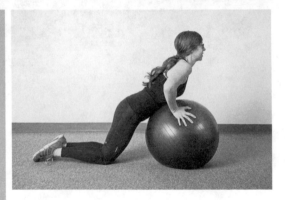

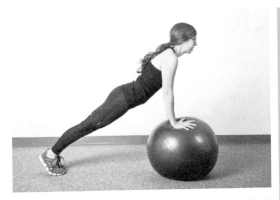

STEP 3

For full push ups, straighten legs to balance on the balls of feet. Lower upper body towards the ball, pause, push back up to start position. Maintain straight line between shoulders and ankles. Do 10–15 repetitions.

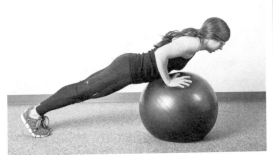

BRIDGE

This is a low-intensity, no-impact exercise targeting the lower body. The addition of the ball engages the core muscles and aids in balance training. Use caution if suffering from peripheral neuropathy.

STEP 1
Sit on ball with feet flat on floor.

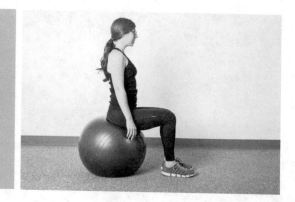

STEP 2
Walk the feet forward until upper body is resting on the ball, with knees bent at 90 degrees. Cross hands over chest.

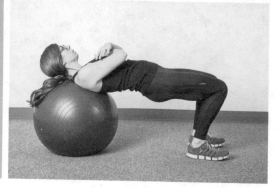

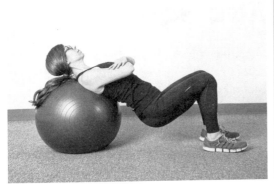

STEP 3
With tight abdominals, lower the hips until just above the floor.

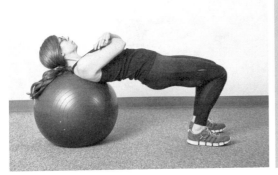

STEP 4
Keeping abdominals firm, press through the heels to lift the hips back to start position. Do 15 repetitions.

LIFT AND SQUEEZE

The lift and squeeze is a moderate-intensity, no-impact exercise. This exercise targets the inner thigh muscles that aid in maintaining knee and hip alignment. The core muscles are also challenged while doing this exercise. This exercise is safe for all fitness levels.

STEP 1
Lie flat on back with feet on either side of stability ball.

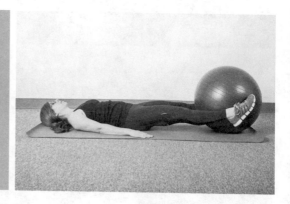

STEP 2
Squeeze the feet against ball and lift off the ground. Keep lower back pressing into floor or mat, abdominals pulled in.

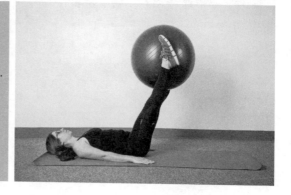

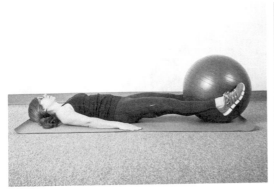

STEP 3
Keeping the feet squeezed against ball, slowly lower back to ground. Do 10–15 repetitions.

AB ROLL

This is a moderate-intensity activity targeting the abdominal muscles. Ab rolls can put some strain on the back and knees, so avoid this exercise if any pain occurs.

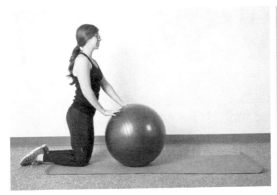

STEP 1
Kneel on floor in front of ball with hands resting on the ball. Keep your elbows bent and hands parallel.

STEP 2

Tightening abdominals, roll ball as far forward as comfortable, keeping knees on floor. Keep spine straight. Do not let hips drop.

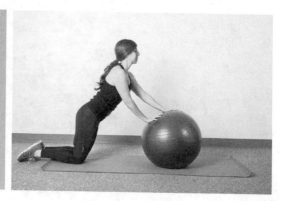

STEP 3

Pause in rolled out position for one deep breath. Slowly roll back to start. Do 10–15 repetitions.

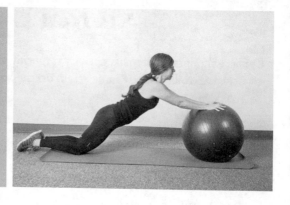

LEG EXTENSIONS

Leg extensions on a stability ball are a double duty strength and balance exercise. This exercise targets the thigh muscles as well as the core. It is a low-intensity, no-impact exercise that is safe for all fitness levels.

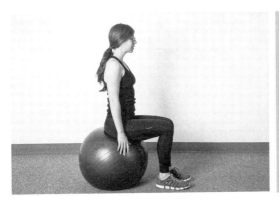

STEP 1
Sit on ball with feet flat on floor. Place hands on either side of ball for stability.

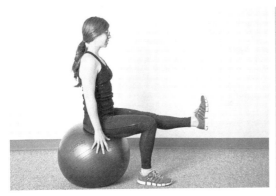

STEP 2
Sitting tall, lift left leg straight out, toes pointing to ceiling.

STEP 3
Lower to start position. Do 10–15 repetitions. Repeat with other leg.

STEP 4
Lift arms off ball to create a greater balance challenge.

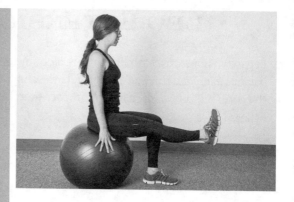

KNEE LIFTS

Knee lifts on a stability ball target the hip muscles as well as the core and back. This exercise is low intensity and is a double duty exercise that helps not only strength but also balance and posture. This exercise is safe for all fitness levels.

STEP 1
Sit on ball with feet flat on floor. Place hands on either side of ball for stability.

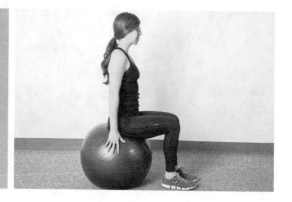

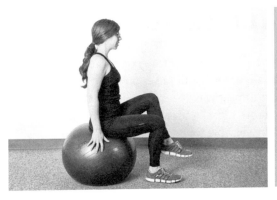

STEP 2
Sit tall with abdominals tight. Lift knee as high as possible. Do not round forward, but keep a long spine.

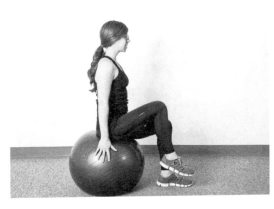

STEP 3
Lower to start position. Do 10–15 reps. Repeat with other leg.

STEP 4
Lift arms off ball to create greater balance challenge.

CALF RAISES

Strong calves are an important element for good balance and proper knee and ankle alignment. Calf raises on the stability ball are a low-intensity, low-impact way to strengthen the calf muscles while also working the core muscles and improving posture. This exercise may not be suitable for people with peripheral neuropathy in the feet.

STEP 1
Sit on the ball with feet at hip distance (feet together for increased balance challenge). Keep spine long and abdominals pulled in.

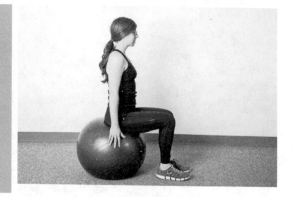

STEP 2
Lift right heel off ground, pause. Lower to start position. Do 10–15 repetitions. Repeat with other leg.

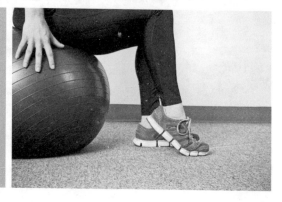

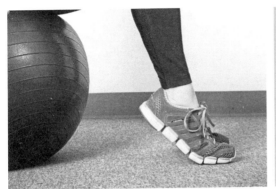

STEP 3
For added challenge, do both legs.

BICEP CURLS

This is a low-intensity, no-impact exercise. Bicep curls target the muscle on the front of the front of the arm. This muscle is important for lifting and pulling. The addition of the ball helps with core strength and balance. If hand strength is compromised because of neuropathy of the hand, use caution. This exercise can also be done with wrist weights. Do one arm at a time to decrease the challenge, if needed.

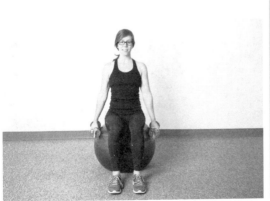

STEP 1
Sit on ball with feet at hip distance (feet closer together for added balance challenge). Keep spine long and abdominals pulled in. Hold a 5–10 lb weight in each hand, palms facing in.

STEP 2

Keeping elbows close to body, curl hands toward shoulders, turning palms up to ceiling. Do 10–15 repetitions.

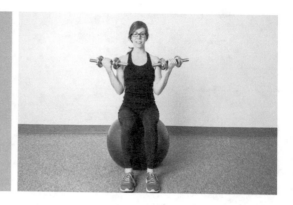

CHEST FLY

Chest fly strengthen the muscles in the front of the chest. These muscles are key muscles for good posture. This exercise is a moderate-intensity, no-impact exercise and is safe for all fitness levels. The addition of the ball incorporates core strength and balance.

STEP 1

Sit on ball, feet at hip distance. Hold a 5–10 lb weight in each hand. Walk feet forward until upper back is resting on ball. Keep hips lifted.

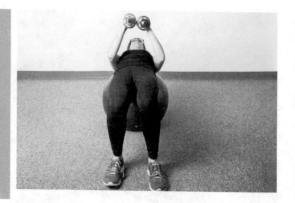

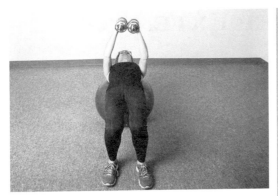

STEP 2
Straighten arms over head so hands are directly over the face, palms in. Arms should be nearly straight, keeping slight bend in elbow.

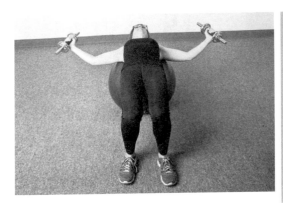

STEP 3
Lower arms out to sides, keeping elbows slightly bent.

STEP 4
Return to start position. Do 10–15 repetitions.

TRICEP EXTENSION

This is a low-intensity, no-impact exercise. Tricep extensions
work the back of the arms, strengthening the muscles in charge
of pulling and pressing. The addition of the ball incorporates core
strength and balance.

STEP 1
Sit on ball, feet at
hip distance. Hold
a 5–10 lb weight
in each hand.

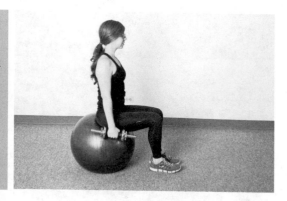

STEP 2
Walk feet forward
until upper back
is resting on ball.
Keep hips lifted.

STEP 3
Straighten arms
overhead so hands
are directly over
the face, palms in.
Arms should be
straight.

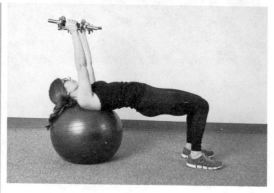

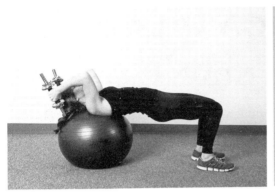

STEP 4
Bend elbows to 90 degrees, lowering hands behind head.

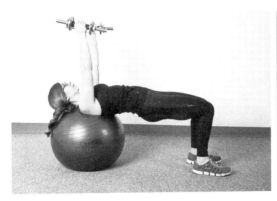

STEP 5
Press back to start position. Do 10–15 repetitions.

YOGA POSES

MOUNTAIN POSE

Mountain Pose is a low-intensity pose that is safe for all fitness levels. This exercise is beneficial for improving posture and lower body strength, as well as, strengthening the core.

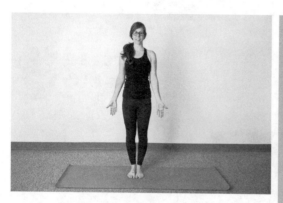

STEP 1
Stand tall with feet at hip distance. Tuck tail bone in and pull abdominals in toward spine. Relax shoulders; let arms hang by sides with palms facing out.

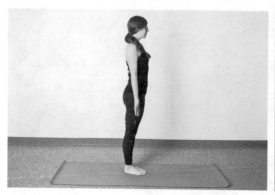

STEP 2
Reach crown of head toward the ceiling while pushing heels down into floor. Hold for 5 breaths.

LOW LUNGE/HIGH LUNGE

Low Lunge is a low-intensity balance pose. This pose may be difficult for people with peripheral neuropathy, so practice with caution. Low Lunge strengthens the lower body as well as relieving pressure caused by sciatica. High Lunge is a moderate intensity balance pose that aids in stretching the groin and strengthens the legs.

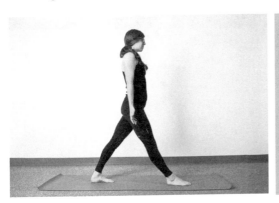

STEP 1
Begin in Mountain Pose. Step left foot back into a wide leg stance.

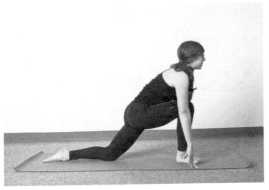

STEP 2
Bend right knee to 90 degrees while lowering left knee to floor. Straighten left leg as much as possible, pressing hips down toward floor.

STEP 3

Place both hands on right knee and straighten upper body. Inhale while sweeping both hands up to the ceiling. For an added balance challenge, look up. Hold for 3 deep breaths. Repeat with right leg.

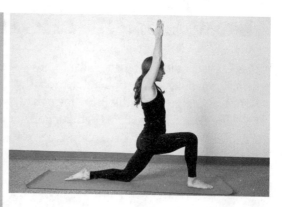

STEP 4

To move into High Lunge, place hand on floor for stability and press left leg straight. Repeat steps 2 and 3.

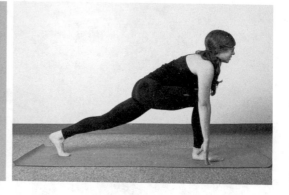

DOWNWARD FACING DOG

Downward Facing Dog is a moderate-intensity pose. It strengthens and stretches muscles of the entire body and aids in preventing osteoporosis. Benefits include improved digestion and increased energy. Be cautious practicing this pose if carpal tunnel syndrome is present.

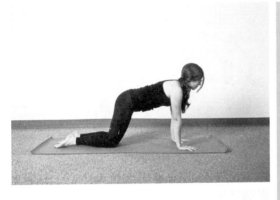

STEP 1
Begin on hands and knees with wrists under shoulders and knees under hips.

STEP 2
Curling toes under, press hips up to ceiling.

STEP 3
Adjust body so arms are straight with palms pressing firmly into floor.

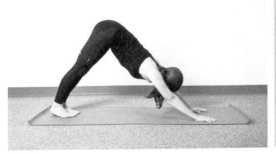

STEP 4
Continue to lift hips up while pressing heels down. Bend knees slightly if pain is felt in legs. Hold for 5 breaths.

WARRIOR POSE

Warrior Pose is a moderate-intensity pose designed to strengthen and stretch the legs and ankles. This pose also facilitates core strengthening and balance training. If problems with the neck are present do not turn to look over the fingertips, but keep head forward.

STEP 1
Begin in Mountain Pose. Step feet into wide leg stance, about 3–4 feet apart.

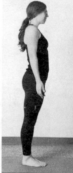 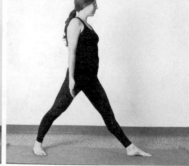

STEP 2
Turn right foot and knee outward, while left foot remains in place.

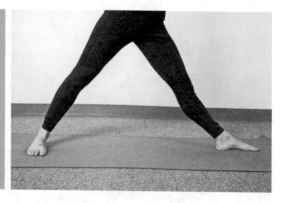

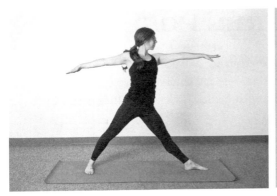

STEP 3
Inhale to sweep arms out to sides and look over fingertips.

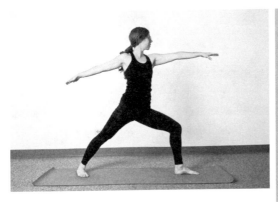

STEP 4
Bend front leg to 90 degrees. Keep upper body very tall.

STEP 5
Keeping back leg very straight, push outside edge of back foot into floor. Hold for 3 breaths.

TREE POSE

This pose is a moderate-intensity balance pose. Tree Pose strengthens the ankles, calves, and thighs. It also promotes strengthening of the core and back. Tree is a balance pose which helps to improve focus.

STEP 1
Begin in Mountain Pose. Rest bottom of right foot against left ankle with knee turned out. If turning knee out causes pain in hip, keep knee pointing forward.

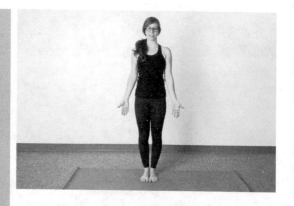

STEP 2
Keep spine long and abdominals firm. Pull right foot up to shin or thigh. Do not rest foot against knee. Reach both hands up to ceiling. Hold for 3 deep breaths. Repeat with other leg.

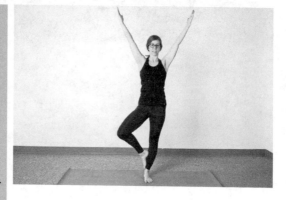

MOON POSE

Moon pose is a low-intensity pose used to stretch the arms and the sides of the waist.

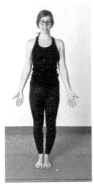 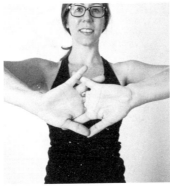

STEP 1
Begin in Mountain Pose. Interlace fingers and turn palms down.

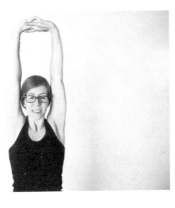

STEP 2
Inhale hands up over head, palms facing up.

STEP 3

With hands reaching up, lean upper body to the right. Hold for 3 deep breaths.

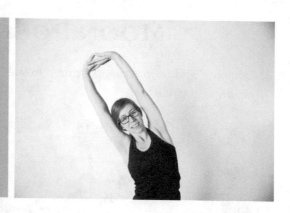

STEP 4

Repeat on left side.

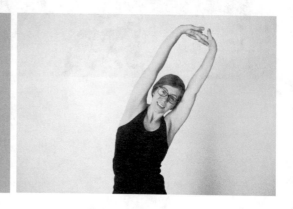

CAT/COW

This flow series is low intensity and aids in strengthening and stretching the low back and core muscles. Cat and Cow is a pose used to practice pairing breath with movement, which helps relive anxiety. Because this pose is done on hands and knees, be cautious if knee or wrist pain occurs.

ON A MAT

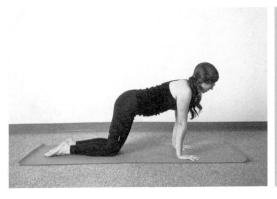

STEP 1
Begin on hands and knees, with wrists under shoulders and knees under hips.

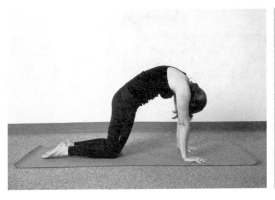

STEP 2
Inhale while rounding the back.

STEP 3

Exhale while pressing hands and knees into floor, arching back, and looking up to ceiling. Each breath pattern equals one set. Continue for 5 sets.

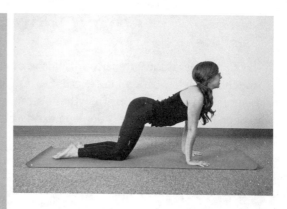

IN A CHAIR

STEP 1

Begin seated in chair with hands on thighs.

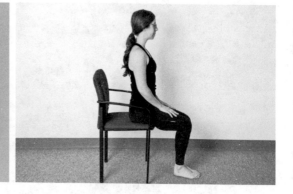

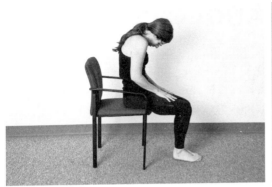

Inhale while
rounding the back.

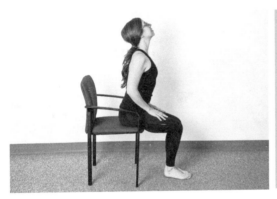

STEP 3

Exhale while
arching back and
looking up to
ceiling. Each
breath pattern
equals one set.
Continue for
5 sets.

TRIANGLE POSE

Triangle Pose is a moderate-intensity pose that stretches and strengthens the lower body. It is also helpful in relieving anxiety and stress. If neck pain occurs in this stretch, do not look up at ceiling, but keep head pointing forward.

STEP 1
Begin in Mountain Pose. Step feet into wide leg stance, about 3–4 feet apart. Position feet as shown here.

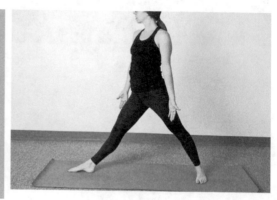

STEP 2
Inhale arms out to sides.

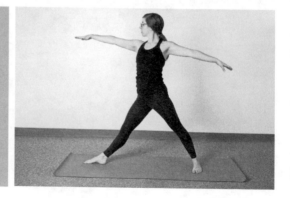

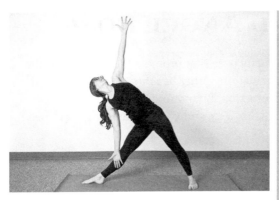

STEP 3

Exhale to reach right hand to shin or ankle. Left arm reaches up to the ceiling. If it's comfortable, turn the head to look up at left arm. Keep back straight, tailbone tucked under.

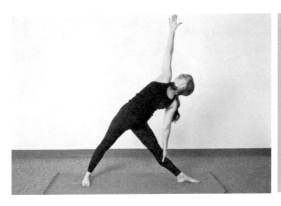

STEP 4

Hold for 3 deeps breaths, then repeat on other side.

BOUND ANGEL POSE

This pose is a low-intensity pose that promotes stimulation of the heart and improves circulation. Other benefits include decreased stress, anxiety, and depression. Bound Angel Pose focuses on stretching the inner thigh, groin, and knees. If hip, groin, or knee pain is present, sit up on a pillow or yoga block.

STEP 1
Sit tall with feet flat on floor, knees bent.

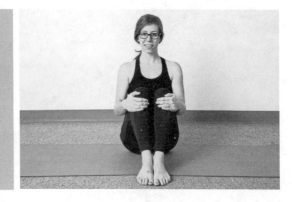

STEP 2
Open knees out to sides and pull heels in toward pelvis.

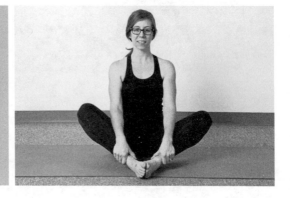

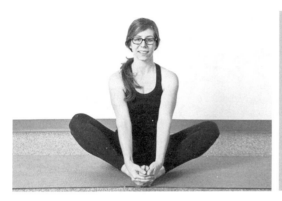

STEP 3
Place hands
around feet.

STEP 4
Round forward,
bringing head
towards feet. Hold
for 3 deep breaths.

BOAT POSE

Boat Pose is a moderate-intensity strengthener for the abdomen,
hips, and spine. This pose stimulates digestion and aids in stress
relief. If neck pain or injury is present, do this pose close enough
to a wall to rest the back of the head against it.

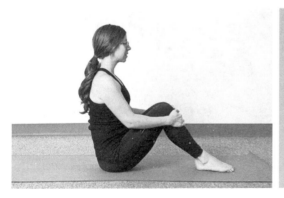

STEP 1
Sit tall with knees
bent, feet flat on
floor. Place hands
behind knees.

STEP 2
Keeping abdominals firm, rock back onto tailbone. Lift feet up until calves are parallel to floor.

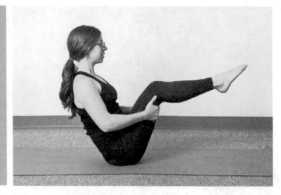

STEP 3
Reach arms straight forward.

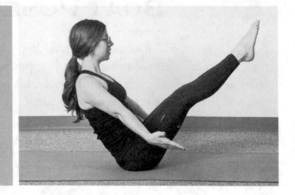

COBRA POSE

Cobra Pose is a moderate-intensity pose that aids in strengthening the spine and the back of the legs. Cobra also helps to relieve symptoms of sciatica. It is considered therapeutic for asthma suffers, as it opens up the heart and lungs. Avoid this pose if back injury or back pain is present.

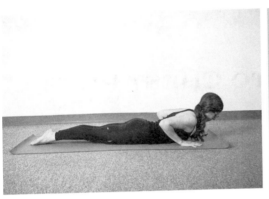

STEP 1
Lie on stomach, hands under shoulders, legs outstretched, tops of feet on floor.

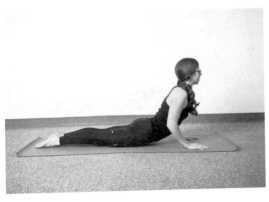

STEP 2
Pull the abdominals in toward spine, tucking tailbone in. Begin to curl upper body off of floor, straightening arms and arching spine.

STEP 3
Keep a slight bend in elbows.

STEP 4
Legs remain straight, hips pressing into floor. Hold for 3 deep breaths.

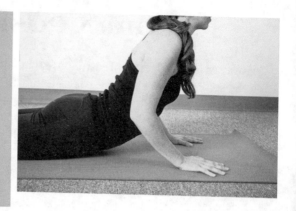

KNEE TO CHEST POSE

This is a low-intensity pose that aids in stretching the low back muscles and the groin. Knee to Chest Pose also promotes deep breathing and relaxation.

STEP 1
Lie on back, legs flat on floor.

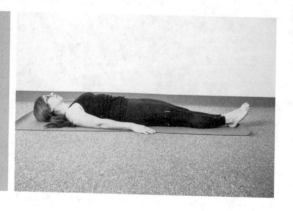

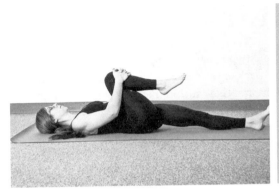

STEP 2
Pull right knee into chest. Press back of head and tailbone into floor. Hold for 5 deep breaths.

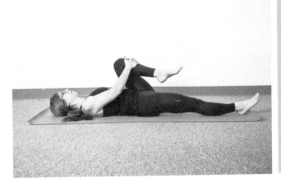

STEP 3
Repeat with left leg.

STAFF POSE

This pose is a low-intensity pose. It is designed to stretch the back and shoulders and the back of the legs. Staff Pose is a great pose to aid in improving posture. Use caution if low back pain or injury is present.

STEP 1

Sit up tall, legs outstretched, feet flexed. Inhaling, reach hands up over head.

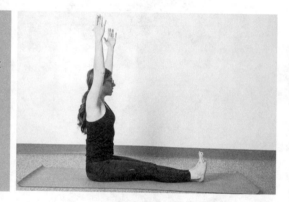

STEP 2

Exhaling, hinge forward, reaching hands towards feet. Keep spine long. Hold for 5 deep breaths.

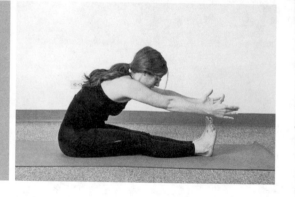

CHILD'S POSE

Child's Pose is a low-intensity pose designed to relieve stres.
fatigue. This pose stretches the back, hips, and ankles. It can
aid in relieving back and neck pain. Avoid this pose if knee inj
is present.

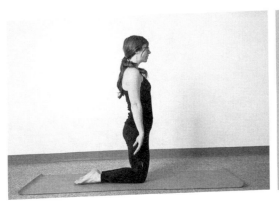

STEP 1
Sit on knees, big toes touching.

STEP 2
Lower hips onto heels and abdominals onto thighs.

STEP 3
Rest forehead on floor or pillow. Reach hands back toward feet. Hold for 5 deep breaths.

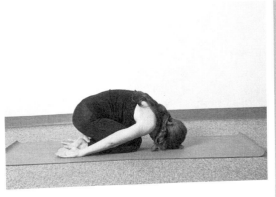

‎PSE POSE

‎...y pose traditionally used at the end
‎... pose relaxes the body, aiding in re-
‎...ure. Corpse Pose also reduces stress and
‎...as improving sleep patterns.

1
‎...at on back
‎...ms and legs
‎fully outstretched.
Relax back of neck
and lower back.

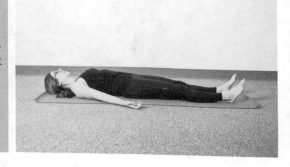

STEP 2
Let hands and feet
fall naturally to
the sides. Breathe
deeply. Hold for 5
minutes.

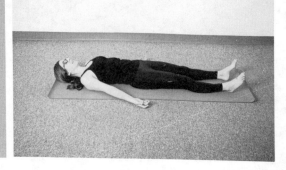

KEEPING AN EXERCISE LOG

As you take control of your diabetes, one of your most valuable tools is knowledge: knowledge of diabetes, knowledge of food and how it interacts with your body, and knowledge of your blood sugar. The more you track your blood sugar, the better your control over it will be.

But tracking your blood sugar alone doesn't give you the whole story. You can give yourself—and your health care team—a fuller picture of what's going on with your body when you track not only your blood sugar, but also your food intake, your mood, and your exercise regimen. That way, you can look back and spot patterns. You can see how a particular food caused a spike in your blood sugar, or how a particular form of exercise brought it down quite low. For those reasons, we recommend you keep an exercise log. On the following page, e've provided a template you can use to guide you, but as you establish your own routines, you'll begin to note which information you find most helpful, and in what form.

Date/day of the week:_____

Time of day: _____

My warm-up and cool-down:

_____

_____

What I did (activity, intensity, and duration):

_____

_____

How I felt:

_____

_____

<u>Blood sugar</u>
Before exercise   [   ]
During exercise [   ]   Heart rate [   ]
After exercise   [   ]

My medication or insulin intake:

_____

_____

Other notes:

_____

_____